This Medical Journal Belongs To:

_____

_____

_____

CONTACTS

Name	Address	Phone	Email

MEDICAL HISTORY

Name: Birthdate:

Known Allergies: Blood Type:

Family Doctor   Contact:

Medications:

Date	Medical History	Notes

MEDICAL HISTORY

Name: Birthdate:

Known Allergies: Blood Type:

Family Doctor   Contact:

Medications:

Date	Medical History	Notes

INSURANCE

Health Insurance

Dental Insurance

Additional Insurance

Notes

Other

Allergies

Blood Type

DOCTORS

FAMILY DOCTOR
Name:
Address:
Phone:
Additional Info:

FAMILY DENTIST
Name:
Address:
Phone:
Additional Info:

OPTOMETRIST
Name:
Address:
Phone:
Additional Info:

PEDIATRICIAN
Name:
Address:
Phone:
Additional Info:

VETERINARIAN
Name:
Address:
Phone:
Additional Info:

DOCTORS

FAMILY DOCTOR
Name:
Address:
Phone:
Additional Info:

FAMILY DENTIST
Name:
Address:
Phone:
Additional Info:

OPTOMETRIST
Name:
Address:
Phone:
Additional Info:

PEDIATRICIAN
Name:
Address:
Phone:
Additional Info:

VETERINARIAN
Name:
Address:
Phone:
Additional Info:

ANNUAL WELLNESS

YEAR: _____

JANUARY

FEBRUARY

MARCH

APRIL

MAY

JUNE

JULY

AUGUST

SEPTEMBER

OCTOBER

NOVEMBER

DECEMBER

NOTES:

DOCTOR VISITS

Date: Follow Up:

Doctor:

Hospital:

Purpose:

Notes:

Date: Follow Up:

Doctor:

Hospital:

Purpose:

Notes:

DOCTOR VISITS

Date: Follow Up:

Doctor:

Hospital:

Purpose:

Notes:

Date: Follow Up:

Doctor:

Hospital:

Purpose:

Notes:

DOCTOR VISITS

Date: Follow Up:

Doctor:

Hospital:

Purpose:

Notes:

Date: Follow Up:

Doctor:

Hospital:

Purpose:

Notes:

TEST RESULTS

DATE	TEST	DOCTOR	PURPOSE	RESULTS

TEST RESULTS

DATE	TEST	DOCTOR	PURPOSE	RESULTS

SYMPTOMS TRACKER

DATE	DESCRIPTION	DR. VISIT	TREATMENT
		☐	☐
		☐	☐
		☐	☐
		☐	☐
		☐	☐
		☐	☐
		☐	☐
		☐	☐
		☐	☐
		☐	☐
		☐	☐
		☐	☐
		☐	☐
		☐	☐
		☐	☐
		☐	☐
		☐	☐
		☐	☐
		☐	☐
		☐	☐
		☐	☐
		☐	☐
		☐	☐
		☐	☐

SYMPTOMS TRACKER

DATE DESCRIPTION DR. VISIT TREATMENT

ILLNESS TRACKER

DATE	DESCRIPTION	DR. VISIT	TREATMENT
		☐	☐
		☐	☐
		☐	☐
		☐	☐
		☐	☐
		☐	☐
		☐	☐
		☐	☐
		☐	☐
		☐	☐
		☐	☐
		☐	☐
		☐	☐
		☐	☐
		☐	☐
		☐	☐
		☐	☐
		☐	☐
		☐	☐
		☐	☐
		☐	☐

ILLNESS TRACKER

DATE	DESCRIPTION	DR. VISIT	TREATMENT
		☐	☐
		☐	☐
		☐	☐
		☐	☐
		☐	☐
		☐	☐
		☐	☐
		☐	☐
		☐	☐
		☐	☐
		☐	☐
		☐	☐
		☐	☐
		☐	☐
		☐	☐
		☐	☐
		☐	☐
		☐	☐
		☐	☐
		☐	☐
		☐	☐
		☐	☐
		☐	☐

MEDICATIONS

MEDICATION　　　　**USED FOR**　　　　**DOSE**　　　　**TIMES PER DAY:**

MEDICATIONS

MEDICATION	USED FOR	DOSE	TIMES PER DAY:

SURGERIES

DATE	DOCTOR	REASON	RESULTS

IMMUNIZATIONS

DATE: TYPE: PURPOSE: DOCTOR:

PASSWORDS

Website	
Username	
Password	
Email	
Notes	

Website	
Username	
Password	
Email	
Notes	

Website	
Username	
Password	
Email	
Notes	

Website	
Username	
Password	
Email	
Notes	

Website	
Username	
Password	
Email	
Notes	

Website	
Username	
Password	
Email	
Notes	

Website	
Username	
Password	
Email	
Notes	

Website	
Username	
Password	
Email	
Notes	

Health & Self Care Journal

Week of

Monday

Tuesday

Wednesday

Thursday

Friday

Saturday

Sunday

Health & Self Care Journal

Week of

Monday

Tuesday

Wednesday

Thursday

Friday

Saturday

Sunday

Health & Self Care Journal

Week of

Monday

Tuesday

Wednesday

Thursday

Friday

Saturday

Sunday

Health & Self Care Journal

Week of

Monday

Tuesday

Wednesday

Thursday

Friday

Saturday

Sunday

Health & Self Care Journal

Week of

Monday

Tuesday

Wednesday

Thursday

Friday

Saturday

Sunday

Health & Self Care Journal

Week of

Monday

Tuesday

Wednesday

Thursday

Friday

Saturday

Sunday

Health & Self Care Journal

Week of

Monday

Tuesday

Wednesday

Thursday

Friday

Saturday

Sunday

Health & Self Care Journal

Week of

Monday

Tuesday

Wednesday

Thursday

Friday

Saturday

Sunday

Health & Self Care Journal

Week of

Monday

Tuesday	Wednesday

Thursday

Friday

Saturday

Sunday

Health & Self Care Journal

Week of

Monday

Tuesday

Wednesday

Thursday

Friday

Saturday

Sunday

Health & Self Care Journal

Week of

Monday

Tuesday

Wednesday

Thursday

Friday

Saturday

Sunday

Health & Self Care Journal

Week of

Monday

Tuesday

Wednesday

Thursday

Friday

Saturday

Sunday

Health & Self Care Journal

Week of

Monday

Tuesday

Wednesday

Thursday

Friday

Saturday

Sunday

Health & Self Care Journal

Week of

Monday

Tuesday

Wednesday

Thursday

Friday

Saturday

Sunday

Health & Self Care Journal

Week of

Monday

Tuesday

Wednesday

Thursday

Friday

Saturday

Sunday

Health & Self Care Journal

Week of

Monday

Tuesday

Wednesday

Thursday

Friday

Saturday

Sunday

Health & Self Care Journal

Week of

Monday

Tuesday

Wednesday

Thursday

Friday

Saturday

Sunday

Health & Self Care Journal

Week of

Monday

Tuesday

Wednesday

Thursday

Friday

Saturday

Sunday

Health & Self Care Journal

Week of

Monday

Tuesday

Wednesday

Thursday

Friday

Saturday

Sunday

Health & Self Care Journal

Week of

Monday

Tuesday

Wednesday

Thursday

Friday

Saturday

Sunday

Health & Self Care Journal

Week of

Monday

Tuesday

Wednesday

Thursday

Friday

Saturday

Sunday

Health & Self Care Journal

Week of

Monday

Tuesday

Wednesday

Thursday

Friday

Saturday

Sunday

Health & Self Care Journal

Week of

Monday

Tuesday

Wednesday

Thursday

Friday

Saturday

Sunday

Health & Self Care Journal

Week of

	Monday

Tuesday	Wednesday

Thursday

Friday

Saturday

Sunday

Health & Self Care Journal

Week of

Monday

Tuesday

Wednesday

Thursday

Friday

Saturday

Sunday

Health & Self Care Journal

Week of

Monday

Tuesday

Wednesday

Thursday

Friday

Saturday

Sunday

Health & Self Care Journal

Week of

Monday

Tuesday

Wednesday

Thursday

Friday

Saturday

Sunday

Health & Self Care Journal

Week of

Monday

Tuesday

Wednesday

Thursday

Friday

Saturday

Sunday

Health & Self Care Journal

Week of

Monday

Tuesday

Wednesday

Thursday

Friday

Saturday

Sunday

Health & Self Care Journal

Week of

Monday

Tuesday

Wednesday

Thursday

Friday

Saturday

Sunday

Health & Self Care Journal

Week of

	Monday

	Tuesday		Wednesday

Thursday

Friday

Saturday

Sunday

Health & Self Care Journal

Week of

Monday

Tuesday

Wednesday

Thursday

Friday

Saturday

Sunday

Health & Self Care Journal

Week of

Monday

Tuesday

Wednesday

Thursday

Friday

Saturday

Sunday

Health & Self Care Journal

Week of

Monday

Tuesday	Wednesday

Thursday

Friday

Saturday

Sunday

Health & Self Care Journal

Week of

Monday

Tuesday

Wednesday

Thursday

Friday

Saturday

Sunday

Health & Self Care Journal

Week of

Monday

Tuesday

Wednesday

Thursday

Friday

Saturday

Sunday

Health & Self Care Journal

Week of

Monday

Tuesday

Wednesday

Thursday

Friday

Saturday

Sunday

Health & Self Care Journal

Week of

Monday

Tuesday

Wednesday

Thursday

Friday

Saturday

Sunday

Health & Self Care Journal

Week of

Monday

Tuesday

Wednesday

Thursday

Friday

Saturday

Sunday

Health & Self Care Journal

Week of

Monday

Tuesday

Wednesday

Thursday

Friday

Saturday

Sunday

Health & Self Care Journal

Week of

Monday

Tuesday

Wednesday

Thursday

Friday

Saturday

Sunday

Health & Self Care Journal

Week of

Monday

Tuesday	Wednesday

Thursday

Friday

Saturday

Sunday

Health & Self Care Journal

Week of

Monday

Tuesday	Wednesday

Thursday

Friday

Saturday

Sunday

Health & Self Care Journal

Week of

Monday

Tuesday

Wednesday

Thursday

Friday

Saturday

Sunday

Health & Self Care Journal

Week of

Monday

Tuesday

Wednesday

Thursday

Friday

Saturday

Sunday

Health & Self Care Journal

Week of

Monday

Tuesday

Wednesday

Thursday

Friday

Saturday

Sunday

Health & Self Care Journal

Week of

Monday

Tuesday

Wednesday

Thursday

Friday

Saturday

Sunday

Health & Self Care Journal

Week of

Monday

Tuesday

Wednesday

Thursday

Friday

Saturday

Sunday

Health & Self Care Journal

Week of

Monday

Tuesday

Wednesday

Thursday

Friday

Saturday

Sunday

Health & Self Care Journal

Week of

Monday

Tuesday

Wednesday

Thursday

Friday

Saturday

Sunday

Health & Self Care Journal

Week of

| Monday |

| Tuesday | Wednesday |

Thursday

Friday

Saturday

Sunday

Health & Self Care Journal

Week of

Monday

Tuesday

Wednesday

Thursday

Friday

Saturday

Sunday

Made in United States
Troutdale, OR
01/09/2024